The Best Low Sodium Cooking Guide

Easy & Healthy Recipes to Make Unforgettable Low Sodium Courses

Alfred Hopper

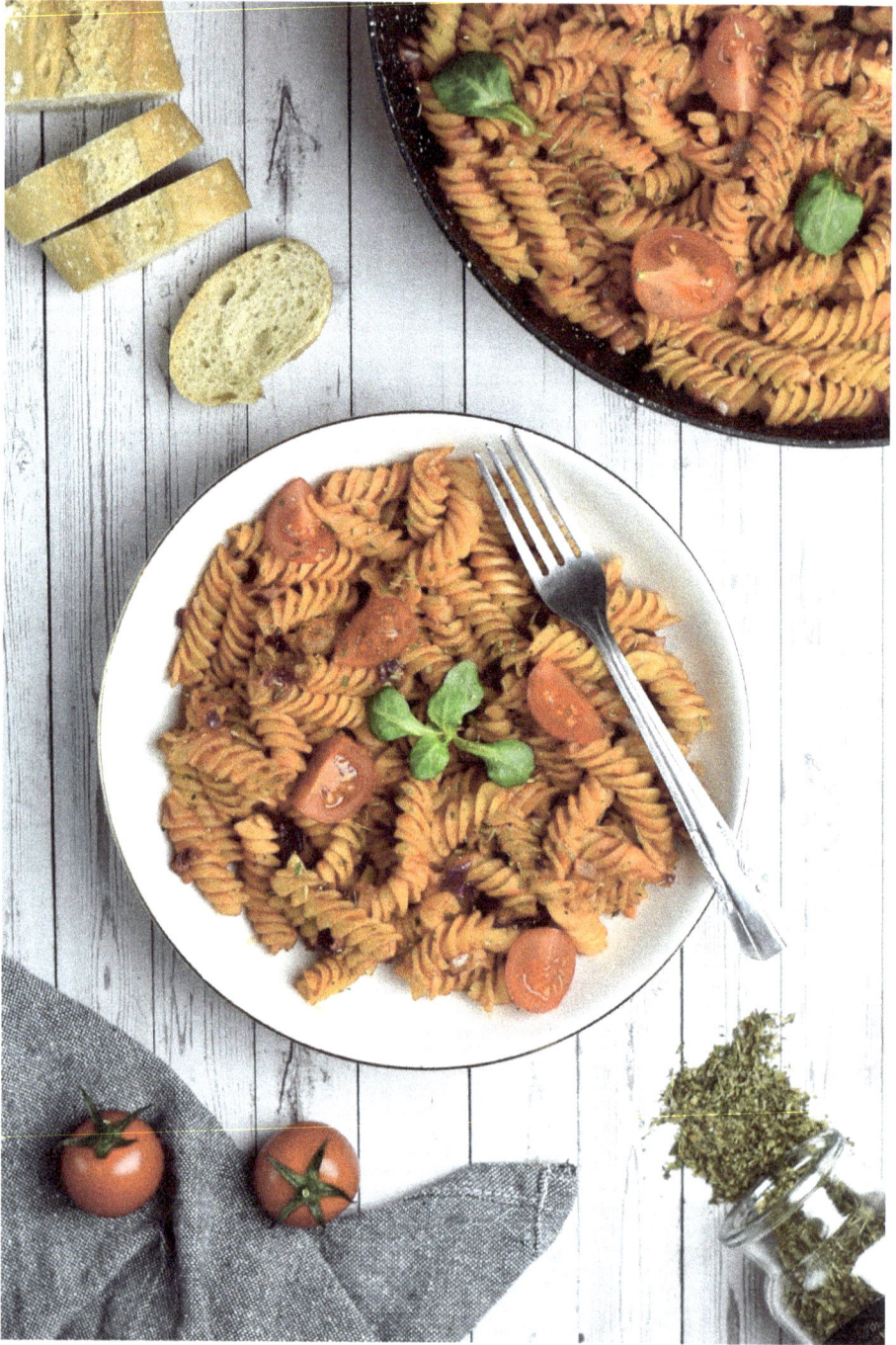

professional advice. The content within this book has been derived from various sources. Please consult a licensed professional before attempting any techniques outlined in this book.

By reading this document, the reader agrees that under no circumstances is the author responsible for any losses, direct or indirect, which are incurred as a result of the use of information contained within this document, including, but not limited to, — errors, omissions, or inaccuracies.

Table of Contents

Vegetables In Warm Citrus Vinaigrette

Servings: 4

Ingredients:

- Pinch saffron
- Pinch grated lemon or lime zest
- 2 teaspoons grapeseed oil
- 1 tablespoon water
- Olive oil spray
- 1 (10-ounce) package frozen California-style vegetables, thawed
- 1 tablespoon frozen orange juice concentrate
- 1/8 teaspoon freshly ground black pepper

Directions:

1. Preheat oven to 350°F.
2. Add the saffron, zest, grapeseed oil, and water to a microwave-safe bowl. Microwave on high for 20–30 seconds, until the water just boils; stir. Cover and set aside to infuse at room temperature while the vegetables bake.
3. Treat an ovenproof casserole dish with the olive oil spray. Add the thawed vegetables.

Spray a light coating of olive oil spray over the top of the vegetables. Cover and bake for 15 minutes. Carefully remove the cover and stir the vegetables. Spray with an additional coating of the olive oil spray. Bake for an additional 15 minutes.

4.   During the last few minutes of the baking time, add the frozen orange juice concentrate to the saffron-oil mixture. Whisk to combine.

5.   Remove the vegetables from the oven. Pour the saffron-orange vinaigrette over the vegetables and add the pepper; toss to combine. Serve immediately.

Nutrition Info: (Per Serving):Calories: 72; Total Fat: 2 g; Saturated Fat: 0 g; Cholesterol: 0 mg; Protein: 2 g; Sodium: 24 mg; Potassium: 149 mg; Fiber: 3 g; Carbohydrates: 10 g; Sugar: 3 g

Spanish Green Beans

Servings: 4

Ingredients:

- ½ pound (225 g) green beans
- ¼ cup (40 g) onion, chopped
- ¼ cup (30 g) green bell pepper, chopped
- 1 tablespoon (15 ml) olive oil
- 1 cup (180 g) tomatoes, chopped
- ½ teaspoon dried basil
- ½ teaspoon dried rosemary

Directions:

1. Cook beans in boiling water until tender. Drain and set aside. Sauté onion and pepper in oil until soft. Add tomatoes and spices. Stir in beans. Heat through.

Nutrition Info: (Per Serving): 53 g water; 43 calories (69% from fat, 5% from protein, 26% from carb); 1 g protein; 3 g total fat; 0 g saturated fat; 3 g monounsaturated fat; 0 g polyunsaturated fat; 3 g carb; 1 g fiber; 2 g sugar; 9 mg calcium; 0 mg iron; 3 mg sodium; 122 mg potassium; 355 IU vitamin A; 13 mg vitamin C; 0 mg cholesterol

Lemon Fingerling Potatoes

Servings: 4

Ingredients:

- 1 pound fingerling potatoes
- 1 cup water
- 2 tablespoons unsalted butter
- 1 tablespoon olive oil
- 3 cloves garlic, minced
- 2 tablespoons lemon juice
- 1/8 teaspoon white pepper

Directions:

1. Wash the potatoes and slice in half lengthwise. Combine in microwave-safe dish with water.
2. Cover and microwave on high for 5–6 minutes or until potatoes are almost tender. Drain well.
3. In large saucepan, melt butter with olive oil over medium heat. Add garlic; cook for 1 minute until fragrant.
4. Carefully add the potatoes; they will splatter a bit, as they are not dry. Cook for 2–4 minutes, shaking pan frequently, until the

potatoes are golden brown and tender. Drizzle with lemon juice, sprinkle with pepper, and serve.

Nutrition Info: (Per Serving):Calories: 186; Total Fat: 9 g; Saturated Fat: 4 g; Cholesterol: 15 mg; Protein: 2 g; Sodium: 14 mg; Potassium: 638 mg; Fiber: 2 g; Carbohydrates: 23 g; Sugar: 1 g

Grilled Vegetable Packs

Servings: 4

Ingredients:

- 2 cups zucchini, sliced
- 2 onions, peeled and sliced
- 2 cups (260 g) carrot, sliced
- ¼ teaspoon black pepper
- ¼ teaspoon garlic powder

Directions:

1. Divide veggies between 4 large squares of aluminum foil. Sprinkle 1 teaspoon of water over each packet. Sprinkle with pepper and garlic. Fold each packet shut and seal well. Grill over medium coals until veggies are tender, about 40 minutes, turning occasionally.

Nutrition Info: (Per Serving): 169 g water; 63 calories (4% from fat, 11% from protein, 85% from carb); 2 g protein; 0 g total fat; 0 g saturated fat; 0 g monounsaturated fat; 0 g polyunsaturated fat; 15 g carb; 4 g fiber; 7 g sugar; 45 mg calcium; 1 mg iron; 52 mg sodium; 459 mg potassium; 7829 IU vitamin A; 18 mg vitamin C; 0 mg cholesterol

Hash Browns With Pear And Apple

Servings: 6

Ingredients:

- 21/2 cups frozen hash brown potatoes, thawed and drained
- 1/3 cup shredded Granny Smith apple
- 1/3 cup shredded pear
- 1 tablespoon lemon juice
- 1 teaspoon dried thyme leaves
- 1/8 teaspoon white pepper
- 3 tablespoons unsalted butter, divided
- 2 tablespoons olive oil

Directions:

1. In large bowl, combine the potatoes, apple, and pear. Sprinkle with lemon juice, thyme, and pepper and mix well. Preheat oven to 300°F.

2. In a large nonstick skillet, melt 2 tablespoons butter and olive oil over medium heat. Drop the potato mixture by 1/2-cup portions into the butter, making 3 patties at a time.

3. Cook, pressing down occasionally with a spatula, until the patties are brown on the

bottom, about 4–6 minutes. Flip carefully with a spatula and cook on the second side until brown, about 3–5 minutes longer. Remove to a baking pan and place in the oven to keep warm. Cook the second batch as you did the first, adding another tablespoon of butter before cooking, and serve immediately.

Nutrition Info: (Per Serving):Calories: 172; Total Fat: 10 g; Saturated Fat: 4 g; Cholesterol: 15 mg; Protein: 2 g; Sodium: 20 mg; Potassium: 273 mg; Fiber: 1 g; Carbohydrates: 18 g; Sugar: 1 g

Oven-fried Potato Wedges

Servings: 4

Ingredients:

- Olive oil spray
- 4 large baking potatoes, washed and cut into 6 wedges each
- 3/4 teaspoon freshly ground black pepper
- 1 teaspoon garlic powder
- 1/2 teaspoon dried rosemary, finely crushed
- 1/2 teaspoon grated lemon zest

Directions:

1. Preheat the oven to 400°F.
2. Spray a baking sheet with the olive spray oil. Arrange the potato wedges on the sheet. Spray the potatoes with a thin layer of the olive oil spray. Sprinkle the potatoes with the pepper, garlic powder, rosemary, and lemon zest.
3. Bake for 30–35 minutes, turning the potatoes to the other cut side after 20 minutes, until the potatoes are lightly browned, crisp outside, and tender inside.

Nutrition Info: (Per Serving):Calories: 290; Total Fat: 0 g; Saturated Fat: 0 g; Cholesterol: 0 mg; Protein: 7 g; Sodium: 41 mg; Potassium: 1,644 mg; Fiber: 6 g; Carbohydrates: 64 g; Sugar: 3 g

Refried Beans

Servings: 8

Ingredients:

- 2 tablespoons olive oil
- 1 medium onion, finely chopped
- 3 cloves garlic, minced
- 1 or 2 jalapeño peppers, finely chopped
- 2 (16-ounce) cans no-salt-added kidney beans, rinsed and drained
- 1 cup Chicken Stock or Vegetable Broth
- 1 tablespoon chili powder
- 1 teaspoon ground cumin
- 2 tablespoons lemon juice
- 1/4 teaspoon black pepper

Directions:

1. In large skillet, heat olive oil over medium heat. Add onion, garlic, and jalapeño pepper; cook and stir for 4–5 minutes until crisp-tender.

2. Add the kidney beans. Mash with a potato masher until the beans are as smooth as you want. You can leave some of the beans whole

for more texture. Add stock or broth, stirring so the beans absorb the liquid.

3.   Simmer for 5 minutes, then add the chili powder, cumin, lemon juice, and pepper and mix well. Use immediately, or cool completely, then freeze in 1 cup measures. To thaw, let stand in refrigerator for several hours.

Nutrition Info: (Per Serving):Calories: 186; Total Fat: 4 g; Saturated Fat: 0 g; Cholesterol: 0 mg; Protein: 10 g; Sodium: 21 mg; Potassium: 526 mg; Fiber: 8 g; Carbohydrates: 27 g; Sugar: 0 g

Stuffing

Servings: 12

Ingredients:

- 6 cups (300 g) Stuffing Bread, cubed or crumbled
- 2 cups (475 ml) low sodium chicken broth or turkey broth
- 1 cup (160 g) onion, chopped
- ½ cup (50 g) celery, chopped
- 2 teaspoons (1.2 g) dried tarragon
- 1 teaspoon dried sage
- 1 teaspoon poultry seasoning
- 1 ½ teaspoons black pepper

Directions:

1. Combine all ingredients and toss lightly. Place in a greased 9 × 13-inch (23 × 33-cm) baking dish. Bake at 350°F (180°C, gas mark 4) until heated through, about 30 minutes.

Nutrition Info: (Per Serving): 64 g water; 71 calories (11% from fat, 15% from protein, 74% from carb); 3 g protein; 1 g total fat; 0 g saturated fat; 0 g monounsaturated fat; 0 g polyunsaturated fat; 13 g carb; 1 g fiber; 2 g sugar; 37 mg calcium; 1 mg iron;

27 mg sodium; 101 mg potassium; 34 IU vitamin A; 1 mg vitamin C; 0 mg cholesterol

Cornbread Stuffing

Servings: 10

Ingredients:

- For cornbread:
- 1 cup (110 g) all-purpose flour
- 2 cups (275 g) cornmeal
- 1 tablespoon (14 g) sodium-free baking powder
- 2 cups (475 ml) buttermilk
- ½ cup (120 ml) canola oil
- For stuffing:
- ½ cup (50 g) celery, chopped
- ½ cup (80 g) onion, chopped
- 1 tablespoon (2 g) dried sage
- ½ tablespoon poultry seasoning
- 1 teaspoon black pepper
- 2 cups (475 ml) low sodium chicken broth or turkey broth

Directions:

1. Preheat oven to 425°F (220°C, gas mark 7). Grease a 12-inch (30-cm) iron skillet or 9 × 9-inch (23 × 23-cm) baking dish and place in oven to heat. Combine cornbread ingredients

In a large bowl and mix well. Pour into hot skillet or dish. Bake until golden brown, about 20 minutes. Crumble corn-bread into large bowl. Add celery, onion, and spices. Stir in enough broth to moisten. Blend well. Spoon into greased 9 × 13-inch (23 × 33-cm) baking dish and bake at 350°F (180°C, gas mark 4) until heated through, about 30 minutes.

Nutrition Info: (Per Serving): 109 g water; 273 calories (39% from fat, 9% from protein, 52% from carb); 6 g protein; 12 g total fat; 1 g saturated fat; 7 g monounsaturated fat; 4 g polyunsaturated fat; 36 g carb; 3 g fiber; 3 g sugar; 139 mg calcium; 2 mg iron; 78 mg sodium; 358 mg potassium; 116 IU vitamin A; 2 mg vitamin C; 2 mg cholesterol

Roasted Cauliflower With Smoked Paprika

Servings: 4–6

Ingredients:

- 1 head cauliflower, broken into small florets
- 3 tablespoons extra-virgin olive oil
- 1 tablespoon smoked paprika
- 1 teaspoon dried marjoram leaves
- 1/2 teaspoon dried thyme leaves
- 1/4 teaspoon pepper
- 2 tablespoons lemon juice

Directions:

1. Preheat oven to 425°F.
2. On a baking sheet with sides, toss cauliflower florets and olive oil. Sprinkle with paprika, marjoram, thyme, pepper, and lemon juice and toss again.
3. Roast cauliflower for 8–12 minutes or until tender and light golden. Remove from oven, transfer to serving bowl, and serve immediately.

Nutrition Info: (Per Serving):Calories: 100; Total Fat: 7 g; Saturated Fat: 0 g; Cholesterol: 0 mg; Protein: 3 g; Sodium: 42 mg; Potassium: 459 mg; Fiber: 4 g; Carbohydrates: 8 g; Sugar: 3 g

Scalloped Potatoes

Servings: 8

Ingredients:

- 6 russet potatoes
- 11/2 cups Slow Cooker Caramelized Onions
- 5 cloves garlic, minced
- 1 cup heavy cream
- 1 cup whole milk
- 1/4 cup Mustard
- 2 tablespoons unsalted butter

Directions:

1. Preheat oven to 350°F. Peel the potatoes and slice them 1/8" thick. As you work, put the sliced potatoes in a bowl of cold water.

2. When all of the potatoes are sliced, dry with a kitchen towel and layer them in a 9" × 13" glass baking dish with the onions and garlic.

3. In medium bowl, combine cream, milk, and mustard and mix with a whisk until blended. Pour slowly over the potatoes. Dot the top with the butter.

4. Bake, covered, for 1 hour. Uncover the potatoes and bake for 25–35 minutes longer or until the potatoes are tender and the top is golden brown.

Nutrition Info: (Per Serving):Calories: 448; Total Fat: 19 g; Saturated Fat: 9 g; Cholesterol: 51 mg; Protein: 9 g; Sodium: 56 mg; Potassium: 1,462 mg; Fiber: 6 g; Carbohydrates: 60 g; Sugar: 8 g

Curried Parsnip Purée

Servings: 4

Ingredients:

- 6 parsnips, peeled and cut into 1/2" cubes
- 1 teaspoon Hot Curry Spice Blend
- 4 teaspoons unsalted butter
- 1/2 cup warm skim milk

Directions:

1. Cook the parsnip cubes in gently boiling water for 12 minutes or until tender. Drain well.

2. Add the parsnips to the bowl of a food processor along with the remaining ingredients; process until smooth.

Nutrition Info: (Per Serving):Calories: 215; Total Fat: 4 g; Saturated Fat: 2 g; Cholesterol: 10 mg; Protein: 4 g; Sodium: 40 mg; Potassium: 932 mg; Fiber: 8 g; Carbohydrates: 42 g; Sugar: 13 g

Roasted And Glazed Root Vegetables

Servings: 4

Ingredients:

- Olive oil spray
- 4 small beets, peeled and diced
- 2 small white turnips, peeled and diced
- 4 large carrots, peeled and sliced
- 2 parsnips, peeled and diced
- 4 cloves garlic, minced
- 1 tablespoon candied ginger, minced
- 4 teaspoons honey
- 1/4 teaspoon (or to taste) freshly ground pepper
- Optional: Chopped watercress, for garnish

Directions:

1. Preheat the oven to 350°F.
2. Spray a jellyroll pan with the olive oil spray. Arrange the vegetables in a single layer across the pan. Sprinkle the garlic and ginger over the vegetables. Spray lightly with the olive oil spray.
3. Bake for 30 minutes. Drizzle the honey over the top of the vegetables. Use a spatula to stir

the vegetables and then spread them back out into a single layer across the pan. Sprinkle with the ground pepper. Bake for an additional 15 minutes or until the vegetables are fork tender.

4. Transfer the vegetables to a serving bowl, stirring well to mix; toss with chopped watercress, if desired.

Nutrition Info: (Per Serving):Calories: 156; Total Fat: 0 g; Saturated Fat: 0 g; Cholesterol: 0 mg; Protein: 3 g; Sodium: 103 mg; Potassium: 761 mg; Fiber: 6 g; Carbohydrates: 37 g; Sugar: 21 g

Caribbean Sweet Potatoes

Servings: 4

Ingredients:

- 2 sweet potatoes, peeled and cubed
- 1 teaspoon vegetable oil
- ¼ cup (30 g) red bell pepper, chopped
- ¼ cup (40 g) onion, chopped
- ¼ cup (60 g) brown sugar
- ¼ cup (60 ml) orange juice
- 2 teaspoons (10 ml) lime juice
- 1 ½ teaspoons Jerk Seasoning

Directions:

1. Cook sweet potatoes in boiling water until just tender. Drain well. Heat oil in large skillet. Add sweet potatoes, bell pepper, and onion to pan and mix well. Combine sugar, juices, and seasoning in a small bowl. Add juice mixture to pan with vegetables and cook over medium heat to reduce liquid until syrupy.

Nutrition Info: (Per Serving): 90 g water; 132 calories (9% from fat, 4% from protein, 88% from carb); 1 g protein; 1 g total fat; 0 g saturated fat; 0 g monounsaturated fat; 1 g polyunsaturated fat; 30 g

carb; 2 g fiber; 18 g sugar; 36 mg calcium; 1 mg iron; 26 mg sodium; 278 mg potassium; 158 IU vitamin A; 25 mg vitamin C; 0 mg cholesterol

Grilled Asparagus

Servings: 4

Ingredients:

- 1 pound asparagus
- 1 tablespoon (15 ml) lemon juice
- 1 tablespoon (15 ml) olive oil
- ¼ teaspoon black pepper, freshly ground

Directions:

1. Trim the asparagus spears and sprinkle with lemon juice and oil. Grind pepper over asparagus. Grill over medium high heat for 3 to 4 minutes, turning once when first side begins to brown in spots.

Nutrition Info: (Per Serving): 109 g water; 54 calories (52% from fat, 17% from protein, 32% from carb); 3 g protein; 4 g total fat; 1 g saturated fat; 3 g monounsaturated fat; 0 g polyunsaturated fat; 5 g carb; 2 g fiber; 2 g sugar; 28 mg calcium; 2 mg iron; 2 mg sodium; 236 mg potassium; 858 IU vitamin A; 8 mg vitamin C; 0 mg cholesterol

Couscous Pilaf

Servings: 4

Ingredients:

- 1 cup unflavored couscous
- 2 cups Chicken Stock or Vegetable Broth
- 2 tablespoons unsalted butter
- 1 tablespoon olive oil
- 1 medium onion, minced
- 1 leek, chopped
- 1/2 cup toasted pine nuts
- 2 tablespoons chopped fresh basil leaves
- 2 tablespoons chopped flat-leaf parsley
- 2 teaspoons chopped fresh mint

Directions:

1. In medium bowl, place couscous. Bring stock to a boil and pour over couscous; cover bowl with a plate and set aside.

2. In large saucepan, melt butter and olive oil over medium heat. Add onion and leek; cook and stir until vegetables are tender, about 7–9 minutes.

3. Uncover couscous and fluff with a fork. Add to the onion mixture along with pine nuts. Cook and stir for 2 minutes.
4. Stir in basil, parsley, and mint and stir to combine. Serve immediately.

Nutrition Info: (Per Serving):Calories: 317; Total Fat: 21 g; Saturated Fat: 5 g; Cholesterol: 15 mg; Protein: 8 g; Sodium: 47 mg; Potassium: 315 mg; Fiber: 2 g; Carbohydrates: 25 g; Sugar: 1 g

Butternut Squash Cheese Muffins

Servings: 12

Ingredients:

- 1 tablespoon unsalted butter
- 1 tablespoon extra-light olive oil or canola oil
- 1 cup chopped sweet onion
- 1 cup sliced button mushrooms
- 1/4 cup water
- 2 cups cubed Roasted Butternut Squash
- 6 tablespoons unbleached all-purpose flour
- 3 tablespoons oat bran or wheat germ
- 2 large eggs
- 1/4 teaspoon freshly ground black pepper
- 1/2 cup grated Jarlsberg cheese
- 1 tablespoon hulled sesame seeds

Directions:

1. Preheat oven to 400°F.
2. Add the butter and oil to a nonstick sauté pan over high heat. When the butter begins to sizzle, reduce heat to medium and add the onion and mushrooms. Sauté until the onion

is transparent, about 4–5 minutes. Set aside to cool.

3.   In the bowl of a food processor or in a blender, combine the cooled sautéed mixture and all of the remaining ingredients except the cheese and sesame seeds; pulse until mixed.

4.   Fold the cheese into the squash mixture. Spoon the resulting batter into muffin cups treated with nonstick spray (or lined with foil muffin liners), filling each muffin cup to the top. Evenly divide the sesame seeds over the top of the batter.

5.   Bake for 35–40 minutes. (For savory appetizers, make 24 mini muffins; bake for 20–25 minutes.)

Nutrition Info: (Per Serving):Calories: 99; Total Fat: 4 g; Saturated Fat: 1 g; Cholesterol: 42 mg; Protein: 4 g; Sodium: 30 mg; Potassium: 142 mg; Fiber: 0 g; Carbohydrates: 10 g; Sugar: 1 g

Curried Chickpeas

Servings: 6

Ingredients:

- 1 tablespoon (11 g) mustard seed
- 1 tablespoon (15 ml) olive oil
- Dash red pepper flakes
- ½ cup (80 g) shallots, minced
- 4 cups (400 g) chickpeas, cooked
- ½ teaspoon turmeric
- ½ teaspoon cumin
- ¼ teaspoon ground ginger
- ¼ cup (15 g) fresh cilantro

Directions:

1. In a large saucepan, fry mustard seeds in oil until they begin to pop. Add the red pepper flakes and shallots and sauté until shallots are soft. Add chickpeas, turmeric, cumin, ginger, and enough water to prevent sticking. Simmer for 15 minutes, sprinkle with cilantro, and serve.

Nutrition Info: (Per Serving): 78 g water; 219 calories (23% from fat, 19% from protein, 59% from carb); 11 g protein; 6 g total fat; 1 g saturated fat; 3 g monounsaturated fat; 2 g polyunsaturated fat; 33 g carb; 9 g fiber; 5 g sugar; 71 mg calcium; 4 mg iron; 11 mg sodium; 393 mg potassium; 309 IU vitamin A; 3 mg vitamin C; 0 mg cholesterol

Zucchini Pudding

Servings: 6

Ingredients:

- 2 cups zucchini, sliced
- 1/2 onion, chopped
- 2 tablespoons (16 g) all-purpose flour
- 1 egg
- 2 tablespoons (10 g) Parmesan cheese, grated
- ½ teaspoon dried oregano
- ⅛ teaspoon garlic powder

Directions:

1. Cook zucchini and onion in boiling water until tender. Combine remaining ingredients. Stir into vegetables. Heat the oven to 350°F (180°C, gas mark 4). Pour the mixture into a greased 1 ½-quart (1 ½-L) baking pan and bake it until it is brown (25 to 35 minutes).

Nutrition Info: (Per Serving): 56 g water; 44 calories (33% from fat, 26% from protein, 41% from carb); 3 g protein; 2 g total fat; 1 g saturated fat; 1 g monounsaturated fat; 0 g polyunsaturated fat; 5 g carb; 1 g fiber; 1 g sugar; 38 mg calcium; 1 mg iron;

50 mg sodium; 143 mg potassium; 145 IU vitamin A; 8 mg vitamin C; 43 mg cholesterol

Stewed Tomatoes

Servings: 6

Ingredients:

- 4 cups (720 g) tomatoes
- 1 onion, chopped
- ¾ cup (75 g) celery, chopped
- ½ cup (60 g) green bell pepper, chopped
- 3 tablespoons (39 g) sugar
- 1 bay leaf
- ⅛ teaspoon black pepper

Directions:

1. Core tomatoes; place in boiling water for 15 to 20 seconds, then place in ice water to cool quickly; peel. Cut tomatoes in wedges. In slow cooker, Combine all ingredients. Cover and cook on low for 8 to 9 hours. Remove bay leaf. Serve as a side dish or freeze in portions for soups or other recipes.

Nutrition Info: (Per Serving): 132 g water; 54 calories (4% from fat, 8% from protein, 88% from carb); 1 g protein; 0 g total fat; 0 g saturated fat; 0 g monounsaturated fat; 0 g polyunsaturated fat; 13 g carb; 2 g fiber; 10 g sugar; 21 mg calcium; 0 mg iron;

18 mg sodium; 315 mg potassium; 918 IU vitamin A; 19 mg vitamin C; 0 mg cholesterol

East Meets West Corn

Servings: 8

Ingredients:

- 2 tablespoons ghee (clarified butter), divided
- 1 teaspoon yellow mustard seeds
- 1/8 teaspoon fenugreek seeds
- 1/4 teaspoon dried red pepper flakes
- 1/4 teaspoon ground ginger
- 1/2 teaspoon asafetida
- 1 large sweet onion, chopped
- 1 medium red bell pepper, seeded and chopped
- 1 medium green bell pepper, seeded and chopped
- 2 cloves garlic, minced
- 1/4 teaspoon turmeric
- 2 jalapeño peppers, seeded and chopped
- 2 (10-ounce) packages frozen sweet corn, thawed
- 2 tablespoons freeze-dried shallot
- 1 teaspoon freeze-dried cilantro
- 21/2 cups plain nonfat yogurt

Directions:

1. Heat a large, deep nonstick sauté pan over medium heat. Melt 1 teaspoon of the ghee. Add the mustard and fenugreek seeds. Cover (because the mustard seeds will pop) and toast for 30 seconds, shaking the pan to move the spices and prevent them from scorching. Transfer to a mortar and pestle along with the red pepper flakes and ginger; pound into a paste. Set aside.

2. Add the remaining ghee to the sauté pan. Add the asafetida and sauté for 1 minute over medium heat. Add the onion and bell peppers; sauté until the onion is transparent. Add the garlic and cook for 1 minute, stirring the garlic into the onion-pepper mixture. Add the turmeric and mustard-seed paste; stir into the onion mixture. (Add 1 or 2 tablespoons of water at this point if the mixture is dry.)

3. Add the jalapeño peppers and corn; stir-fry with the onion-pepper mixture, cooking for 2 minutes. Stir in the shallot, cilantro, and yogurt. Lower the heat and simmer, covered, for 5 minutes. Serve immediately.

Nutrition Info: (Per Serving):Calories: 164; Total Fat: 3 g; Saturated Fat: 2 g; Cholesterol: 9 mg; Protein: 5 g; Sodium: 67 mg; Potassium: 516 mg; Fiber: 9 g; Carbohydrates: 28 g; Sugar: 2 g

Sautéed Spinach And Garlic

Servings: 6

Ingredients:

- 2 (10-ounce) packages baby spinach leaves
- 2 tablespoons olive oil
- 1 tablespoon unsalted butter
- 8 cloves garlic, sliced
- 2 tablespoons lemon juice
- 1 tablespoon honey
- 1/8 teaspoon white pepper
- Pinch nutmeg
- 2 tablespoons toasted sesame seeds

Directions:

1. Rinse the spinach in cold water; it can be very sandy. Don't dry the spinach; just shake off excess water.

2. In a large saucepan with a lid, heat olive oil and butter over medium heat. Add garlic; cook and stir just until the garlic is fragrant, about 1 minute.

3. Add the spinach to pan and toss well with the garlic; cover. Cook for 2 minutes, shaking pan frequently.

4. Remove cover and add lemon juice, honey, pepper, and nutmeg. Cook, stirring frequently, until spinach is wilted, about 1 minute longer. Sprinkle with sesame seeds and serve immediately.

Nutrition Info: (Per Serving):Calories: 111; Total Fat: 8 g; Saturated Fat: 2 g; Cholesterol: 5 mg; Protein: 3 g; Sodium: 76 mg; Potassium: 563 mg; Fiber: 2 g; Carbohydrates: 8 g; Sugar: 3 g

Grilled Corn

Servings: 4

Ingredients:

- ¼ cup (55 g) unsalted butter
- 4 ears corn
- ½ teaspoon black pepper

Directions:

1. Spread the butter on the corn and sprinkle with the pepper. Wrap in heavy-duty aluminum foil and grill until done, about 15 minutes, turning frequently.

Nutrition Info: (Per Serving): 92 g water; 225 calories (45% from fat, 7% from protein, 48% from carb); 4 g protein; 12 g total fat; 7 g saturated fat; 3 g monounsaturated fat; 1 g polyunsaturated fat; 30 g carb; 4 g fiber; 5 g sugar; 10 mg calcium; 1 mg iron; 8 mg sodium; 374 mg potassium; 660 IU vitamin A; 9 mg vitamin C; 31 mg cholesterol

Oven-fried Veggies

Servings: 4

Ingredients:

- 3 slices French Bread , crumbled
- 1 teaspoon dried thyme leaves
- 1 teaspoon paprika
- 1/8 teaspoon white pepper
- 1 cup cauliflower florets
- 1 cup zucchini slices
- 1 cup whole green beans
- 1 small red onion, cut into 1/4" rings
- 1 large egg, beaten
- 1 tablespoon lemon juice
- 2 tablespoons olive oil

Directions:

1. Preheat oven to 425°F. Combine bread crumbs, thyme, paprika, and pepper on a plate. Prepare the vegetables.

2. Combine egg and lemon juice in large bowl. Toss the vegetables in this mixture, then add the bread-crumb mixture and toss until coated.

51

3. Coat a baking sheet with sides with the olive oil. Add the coated vegetables in a single layer.

4. Bake for 14–18 minutes or until the vegetables are golden brown and crisp-tender.

Nutrition Info: (Per Serving):Calories: 165; Total Fat: 8 g; Saturated Fat: 1 g; Cholesterol: 53 mg; Protein: 5 g; Sodium: 45 mg; Potassium: 231 mg; Fiber: 3 g; Carbohydrates: 17 g; Sugar: 1 g

Hush Puppies

Servings: 5

Ingredients:

- 1 cup (140 g) cornmeal
- 1 teaspoon sodium-free baking powder
- ¼ cup (40 g) onion, finely chopped
- ½ tablespoon all-purpose flour
- ½ cup (120 ml) skim milk
- Dash cayenne pepper

Directions:

1. Mix ingredients together. Form into balls and drop into hot oil. Deep-fry until golden brown, about 2 minutes. Drain.

Nutrition Info: (Per Serving): 60 g water; 126 calories (4% from fat, 12% from protein, 84% from carb); 4 g protein; 1 g total fat; 0 g saturated fat; 0 g monounsaturated fat; 0 g polyunsaturated fat; 26 g carb; 3 g fiber; 2 g sugar; 84 mg calcium; 1 mg iron; 17 mg sodium; 266 mg potassium; 1042 IU vitamin A; 57 mg vitamin C; 0 mg cholesterol

Green Bean Casserole

Servings: 6

Ingredients:

- ½ cup (80 g) onion, chopped
- 2 tablespoons (30 ml) vegetable oil
- ¼ cup (60 ml) skim milk
- ⅛ teaspoon pepper
- 10 ounces (280 g) Condensed Cream of Mushroom Soup
- 18 ounces (504 g) frozen green beans
- ½ cup (65 g) French-fried onions

Directions:

1. Sauté onion in oil until tender. Combine all ingredients except French-fried onions in a 1 ½-quart (1 ½-L) casserole. Bake at 350°F (180°C, gas mark 4) for 30 minutes. Sprinkle French-fried onions on top. Bake for 5 minutes longer.

Nutrition Info: (Per Serving): 142 g water; 118 calories (54% from fat, 9% from protein, 37% from carb); 3 g protein; 7 g total fat; 1 g saturated fat; 2 g monounsaturated fat; 4 g polyunsaturated fat; 12 g carb; 3 g fiber; 3 g sugar; 59 mg calcium; 1 mg iron;

36 mg sodium; 241 mg potassium; 628 IU vitamin A; 15 mg vitamin C; 1 mg cholesterol

Creamed Celery And Peas

Servings: 6

Ingredients:

- ⅓ cup (80 ml) water
- 2 cups (200 g) celery, sliced
- 10 ounces (280 g) no-salt-added frozen peas
- ½ cup (115 g) sour cream
- ½ teaspoon dried rosemary
- ⅛ teaspoon garlic powder
- ¼ cup (31 g) slivered almonds

Directions:

1. In a saucepan, bring the water to a boil. Add the celery, cover, and cook for 8 minutes. Add peas and return to boil. Cover and cook for 3 minutes more. Drain. Combine sour cream and spices; mix well. Place vegetables in a serving bowl. Top with sour cream mixture. Sprinkle with almonds.

Nutrition Info: (Per Serving): 104 g water; 212 calories (62% from fat, 14% from protein, 24% from carb); 8 g protein; 15 g total fat; 3 g saturated fat; 8 g monounsaturated fat; 3 g polyunsaturated fat; 13 g

carb; 6 g fiber; 4 g sugar; 105 mg calcium; 2 mg iron; 77 mg sodium; 346 mg potassium; 1299 IU vitamin A; 6 mg vitamin C; 8 mg cholesterol

Sautéed Squash And Zucchini

Servings: 4

Ingredients:

- 1 tablespoon unsalted butter
- 1 tablespoon olive oil
- 1 shallot, minced
- 1 medium zucchini, sliced
- 1 medium yellow summer squash, sliced
- 2 tablespoons lemon juice
- 1 tablespoon minced fresh basil leaves
- 2 tablespoons minced flat-leaf parsley

Directions:

1. Heat butter and olive oil in a large pan over medium heat. Add shallot; cook and stir for 2 minutes or until fragrant.
2. Add the zucchini and squash; cook, stirring frequently, for 5–7 minutes or until tender. Sprinkle with lemon, basil, and parsley, and serve immediately.

Nutrition Info: (Per Serving):Calories: 66; Total Fat: 6 g; Saturated Fat: 2 g; Cholesterol: 7 mg; Protein: 0 g; Sodium: 2 mg; Potassium: 154 mg; Fiber: 0 g; Carbohydrates: 2 g; Sugar: 1 g

Condensed Cream Of Mushroom Soup

Servings: 6

Ingredients:

- 1 cup (70 g) mushrooms, sliced
- ½ cup (80 g) onion, chopped
- 1 tablespoon (0.4 g) dried parsley
- ¼ tablespoon garlic powder
- ½ cup (120 ml) low sodium chicken broth
- ⅔ cup (157 ml) skim milk
- 2 tablespoons (16 g) cornstarch

Directions:

1. Cook mushrooms, onion, and spices in chicken broth until soft. Process in a blender or food processor until well pureed. Shake together milk and cornstarch until dissolved. Cook and stir until thick. Stir in veggie mixture.

Nutrition Info: (Per Serving): 67 g water; 33 calories (6% from fat, 23% from protein, 70% from carb); 2 g protein; 0 g total fat; 0 g saturated fat; 0 g monounsaturated fat; 0 g polyunsaturated fat; 6 g carb; 0 g fiber; 1 g sugar; 44 mg calcium; 0 mg iron;

24 mg sodium; 128 mg potassium; 108 IU vitamin A; 2 mg vitamin C; 1 mg cholesterol

Maple Squash Bake

Servings: 10

Ingredients:

- ¾ cup (83 g) all-purpose flour
- ¾ cup (170 g) brown sugar
- 2 teaspoons (5 g) ground cinnamon
- 1 teaspoon ground allspice
- ½ cup (112 g) unsalted butter
- 1 butternut squash
- ½ cup (50 g) pecans, chopped
- 1 cup (235 ml) maple syrup

Directions:

1. In a bowl, Combine flour, sugar, and spices. Cut in butter until crumbly. Peel squash and cut into ½-inch-thick (1 ¼-cm-thick) slices, removing seeds. Place half of squash in a greased 8 × 8-inch (20 × 20-cm) baking dish. Sprinkle with ½ of the crumb mixture. Repeat layers. Sprinkle pecans on top. Drizzle with maple syrup. Cover with foil. Bake at 350°F (180°C, gas mark 4) for 1 hour. Remove foil. Bake for 10 minutes more.

Nutrition Info: (Per Serving): 14 g water; 301 calories (39% from fat, 2% from protein, 59% from carb); 2 g protein; 13 g total fat; 6 g saturated fat; 5 g monounsaturated fat; 2 g polyunsaturated fat; 46 g carb; 1 g fiber; 35 g sugar; 50 mg calcium; 1 mg iron; 11 mg sodium; 162 mg potassium; 289 IU vitamin A; 0 mg vitamin C; 24 mg cholesterol

Golden Delicious Risotto

Servings: 4

Ingredients:

- 4–5 cups water
- 2 tablespoons extra-virgin olive oil
- 2 tablespoons minced onion or shallot
- 1 cup Arborio rice (short-grain white rice)
- 2 medium-size Golden Delicious apples, peeled, cored, and diced
- 3/4 teaspoon low-sodium chicken base
- 1/4 teaspoon sautéed vegetable base
- 1/3 cup dry white wine
- 2 tablespoons unsalted butter
- 2 tablespoons grated Parmesan cheese
- Optional: Freshly grated nutmeg

Directions:

1. In medium-size saucepan, heat the water to boiling; reduce heat to maintain a steady simmer.

2. In large nonstick sauté pan treated with nonstick spray, bring the olive oil to temperature over medium heat; add the onion (or shallot) and sauté for 3 minutes. Add the

rice and half of the diced apples; sauté, stirring well, for 3 minutes. Add the bases and stir to dissolve. Add the wine and stir until the wine evaporates.

3. Stirring, ladle in enough of the water to just cover the rice (about 3/4 cup). Lower the heat to maintain a steady simmer and cook the rice, stirring constantly, until almost all of the water has been absorbed, about 4 minutes.

4. Continue adding water 1/2 cup at a time, stirring and cooking until absorbed. After 15 minutes, stir in the remaining diced apples. The rice is done when it is creamy yet firm in the center (al dente). Total cooking time will be around 25–30 minutes.

5. Remove pan from heat and stir in the butter and Parmesan cheese. Grate nutmeg over the top of each serving, if desired, and serve immediately.

Nutrition Info: (Per Serving):Calories: 376; Total Fat: 13 g; Saturated Fat: 5 g; Cholesterol: 17 mg; Protein: 5 g; Sodium: 39 mg; Potassium: 125 mg; Fiber: 1 g; Carbohydrates: 55 g; Sugar: 8 g

Black-eyed Peas And Rice

Servings: 4

Ingredients:

- 1 cup (225 g) black-eyed peas
- 4 cups (940 ml) water
- 3 teaspoons (15 ml) low sodium chicken bouillon
- 2 cloves garlic, crushed
- 1 tablespoon (15 ml) vegetable oil
- 1 tablespoon (2 g) cilantro
- 1 tablespoon (0.4 g) dried parsley
- ½ teaspoon black pepper
- 1 onion, chopped
- 1 cup (235 ml) low sodium tomatoes
- 1 cup (195 g) rice, uncooked

Directions:

1. Combine black-eyed peas and water in large saucepan; add bouillon and garlic. Bring black-eyed pea mixture to a boil; reduce heat and stir in oil, cilantro, parsley, and pepper. Cover and simmer for 15 minutes. Stir in onion and tomatoes. Cover and simmer for 15 minutes or until black-eyed peas are almost soft. Stir

in rice; cover. Cook until rice and black-eyed peas are tender, about 20 minutes.

Nutrition Info: (Per Serving): 382 g water; 142 calories (24% from fat, 9% from protein, 68% from carb); 3 g protein; 4 g total fat; 1 g saturated fat; 1 g monounsaturated fat; 2 g polyunsaturated fat; 25 g carb; 3 g fiber; 4 g sugar; 78 mg calcium; 2 mg iron; 78 mg sodium; 382 mg potassium; 458 IU vitamin A; 19 mg vitamin C; 0 mg cholesterol

Curried Couscous

Servings: 8

Ingredients:

- 1 tablespoon unsalted butter
- 1 teaspoon curry powder
- 11/2 cups couscous
- 11/2 cups boiling water
- 1/4 cup plain nonfat yogurt
- 1/4 cup extra-virgin olive oil
- 1 teaspoon white wine vinegar
- 1/4 teaspoon ground turmeric
- 1/4 teaspoon grated lemon zest
- 1 teaspoon freshly ground black pepper
- 1/2 cup diced carrots
- 1/2 cup minced fresh parsley
- 1/2 cup raisins
- 1/4 cup blanched, sliced almonds
- 2 scallions, white and green parts thinly sliced
- 1/4 cup diced red onion
- 11/2 teaspoons Sesame Salt (Gomashio)

Directions:

1. In a small nonstick skillet, melt the butter until sizzling, then add the curry powder. Stir for several minutes, being careful not to burn the butter. Place the couscous in a medium-size bowl. Pour enough of the boiling water into the pan with the sautéed curry powder to mix it with the water and rinse out the pan. Pour that and the remaining boiling water over the couscous. Cover tightly and allow the couscous to sit for 5 minutes. Fluff with a fork.

2. In a medium bowl, mix together the yogurt, olive oil, vinegar, turmeric, lemon zest, and pepper; pour over the fluffed couscous, and mix well.

3. Add the carrots, parsley, raisins, almonds, scallions, red onion, and sesame salt; mix well. Serve at room temperature.

Nutrition Info: (Per Serving):Calories: 208; Total Fat: 11 g; Saturated Fat: 2 g; Cholesterol: 4 mg; Protein: 4 g; Sodium: 115 mg; Potassium: 224 mg; Fiber: 2 g; Carbohydrates: 24 g; Sugar: 6 g

Summer Squash Casserole

Servings: 6

Ingredients:

- 4 zucchini, or yellow squash, sliced
- 1 medium onion, sliced
- 1 tablespoon (14 g) unsalted butter, melted
- ¼ cup (60 g) sour cream
- ⅛ teaspoon paprika
- 2 tablespoons (6 g) chives, chopped
- 2 cups (230 g) low sodium bread crumbs

Directions:

1. Cook squash and onion in water until almost tender. Drain. Stir together butter, sour cream, paprika, and chives. Add drained squash. Place in 1 ½-quart (1 ½-L) baking dish sprayed with nonstick vegetable oil spray. Top with bread crumbs. Bake at 350°F (180°C, gas mark 4) for 20 minutes.

Nutrition Info: (Per Serving): 28 g water; 189 calories (28% from fat, 11% from protein, 61% from carb); 5 g protein; 6 g total fat; 3 g saturated fat; 1 g monounsaturated fat; 1 g polyunsaturated fat; 28 g

carb; 2 g fiber; 3 g sugar; 83 mg calcium; 2 mg iron; 19 mg sodium; 118 mg potassium; 190 IU vitamin A; 2 mg vitamin C; 9 mg cholesterol

Smashed Potatoes With Caramelized Onions And Garlic

Servings: 8

Ingredients:

- 2 pounds small red potatoes, unpeeled
- 3 tablespoons unsalted butter
- 2/3 cup light cream
- 1/3 cup mascarpone cheese
- 1 cup Slow Cooker Caramelized Onions
- 1 head Roasted Garlic , removed from skins
- 1/4 teaspoon white pepper

Directions:

1. Place potatoes in a large pot and cover with cold water. Bring to a simmer over high heat, then reduce heat to low and simmer for 20–30 minutes or until the potatoes are tender when pierced with a fork. Drain well.
2. Return the potatoes to the hot pot and mash coarsely with a potato masher. Beat in the butter, cream, and mascarpone.

3. Stir in the onions, garlic, and pepper and serve immediately, or cover and place in a 300°F oven to keep warm up to 30 minutes.

Nutrition Info: (Per Serving):Calories: 280; Total Fat: 15 g; Saturated Fat: 8 g; Cholesterol: 43 mg; Protein: 6 g; Sodium: 33 mg; Potassium: 768 mg; Fiber: 3 g; Carbohydrates: 31 g; Sugar: 4 g

Roasted Butternut Squash

Servings: 4

Ingredients:

- 1 large butternut squash

Directions:

1. Preheat oven to 350°F. Wash the outside skin of the squash.
2. Place the whole squash on a jellyroll pan or baking sheet. Pierce the skin a few times with a knife. Bake for 1 hour or until tender.
3. Once the squash is cool enough to handle, slice it open, scrape out the seeds, and scrape the squash pulp off of the skin.

Nutrition Info: (Per Serving):Calories: 93; Total Fat: 0 g; Saturated Fat: 0 g; Cholesterol: 0 mg; Protein: 2 g; Sodium: 4 mg; Potassium: 319 mg; Fiber: 0 g; Carbohydrates: 24 g; Sugar: 0 g

Baked Stuffed Tomatoes

Servings: 4

Ingredients:

- 11/4 cups chopped parsley
- 3 small cloves garlic, finely chopped
- Pinch red pepper flakes
- 3/4 cup bread crumbs
- Olive oil spray
- 10 plum tomatoes, cut in half lengthwise and seeded
- 1/2 teaspoon freshly ground black pepper
- 1/4 teaspoon grated lemon zest
- 1/2 cup water

Directions:

1. Preheat oven to 400°F.
2. In the bowl of a food processor, combine the parsley, garlic, red pepper flakes, and bread crumbs; pulse to chop and mix. Set aside.
3. Prepare a casserole dish or baking pan large enough to hold the tomato halves side by side by spraying it with the olive oil spray. Fill the tomato halves with the bread crumb mixture and place them in the dish or pan. Spray a

light layer of the olive oil spray over the tops of the filled tomatoes. Sprinkle the pepper and lemon zest over the top of the bread crumbs.

4.   Add 1/2 cup water to the bottom of the pan. Cover tightly with an aluminum foil tent. Bake for 30–35 minutes or until the tomatoes are tender.

5.   Remove the aluminum foil. Place the pan under the broiler and broil until crisp and slightly browned, about 2 minutes. (Watch closely so the bread crumbs don't burn!)

Nutrition Info: (Per Serving):Calories: 182; Total Fat: 1 g; Saturated Fat: 0 g; Cholesterol: 0 mg; Protein: 7 g; Sodium: 22 mg; Potassium: 326 mg; Fiber: 4 g; Carbohydrates: 38 g; Sugar: 5 g

Chicken Cream Gravy

Servings: 8

Ingredients:

- 2 tablespoons (28 ml) vegetable oil
- ¼ cup (28 g) all-purpose flour
- 2 teaspoons (10 ml) low sodium chicken bouillon
- 2 cups (475 ml) skim milk

Directions:

1. If using pan that chicken was cooked in, drain off remaining oil and discard all but 2 tablespoons (28 ml). Add flour and bouillon and heat and stir until a paste is formed. Add milk and cook and stir until thickened, scraping any drippings from the bottom of the pan.

Nutrition Info: (Per Serving): 55 g water; 70 calories (46% from fat, 16% from protein, 38% from carb); 3 g protein; 4 g total fat; 1 g saturated fat; 1 g monounsaturated fat; 2 g polyunsaturated fat; 7 g carb; 0 g fiber; 0 g sugar; 89 mg calcium; 0 mg iron; 57 mg sodium; 122 mg potassium; 138 IU vitamin A; 1 mg vitamin C; 1 mg cholesterol

Baked Potato Latkes

Servings: 8

Ingredients:

- Olive oil spray
- 4 medium-size potatoes, peeled and grated
- 1 medium-size red onion, finely chopped
- 1/4 teaspoon salt
- 1/8 teaspoon grated lemon zest
- 1/2 teaspoon freshly grated black pepper
- 1 teaspoon freeze-dried chives
- 1 large egg plus 1 large egg white, lightly beaten together
- 1/4 cup unbleached all-purpose flour
- 1 teaspoon canola oil

Directions:

1. Preheat oven to 350°F. Spray a baking sheet with the olive oil spray.
2. Mix together the remaining ingredients. Spoon the batter onto the baking sheet in 8 equal-sized portions, flattening them slightly. Spray the tops of the pancakes with a light coating of the olive oil spray.

3. Bake for 10 minutes or until brown on the bottom. Turn and bake for an additional 5–10 minutes, until evenly browned.

Nutrition Info: (Per Serving):Calories: 103; Total Fat: 1 g; Saturated Fat: 0 g; Cholesterol: 26 mg; Protein: 3 g; Sodium: 92 mg; Potassium: 329 mg; Fiber: 1 g; Carbohydrates: 20 g; Sugar: 1 g

Marinated Black-eyed Peas

Servings: 4

Ingredients:

- 1 ½ cups (150 g) dried black-eyed peas, cooked and drained
- ½ cup (60 g) green bell pepper, chopped
- ½ cup (60 g) red bell pepper, chopped
- 1 clove garlic, minced
- 1 onion, minced
- 3 tablespoons (45 ml) red wine vinegar
- ¼ cup (60 ml) olive oil
- ½ teaspoon dried thyme

Directions:

1. Pour the drained black-eyed peas into a medium-size bowl and add the bell peppers, garlic, and onion. In another bowl, Combine the vinegar, olive oil, and thyme to form the marinade. Pour the marinade over the black-eyed pea mixture, cover with plastic wrap, and refrigerate overnight so that the flavors blend, stirring occasionally.

Nutrition Info: (Per Serving): 97 g water; 188 calories (64% from fat, 4% from protein, 32% from carb); 2 g protein; 14 g total fat; 2 g saturated fat; 10 g monounsaturated fat; 1 g polyunsaturated fat; 15 g carb; 4 g fiber; 4 g sugar; 81 mg calcium; 1 mg iron; 4 mg sodium; 329 mg potassium; 328 IU vitamin A; 29 mg vitamin C; 0 mg cholesterol

Middle Eastern Glazed Carrots

Servings: 4

Ingredients:

- 4 cups sliced carrots
- 2 teaspoons canola oil
- 2 teaspoons unsalted butter
- 1 teaspoon Middle Eastern Spice Blend
- 2 teaspoons granulated sugar
- 1/8 teaspoon freshly ground black pepper

Directions:

1. Put the carrots in a microwave-safe casserole dish. Cover and microwave on high for 3 minutes; turn the dish. Microwave on high for 4 minutes or until the carrots are tender.

2. Bring a large, deep nonstick sauté pan to temperature over medium heat. Add the oil, butter, and spice blend; sauté the spices for 1 minute.

3. Add the carrots and stir to mix. Sprinkle the sugar and pepper over the carrots and stir-fry until the carrots are heated through and the sugar forms a glaze.

Nutrition Info: (Per Serving):Calories: 95; Total Fat: 4 g; Saturated Fat: 1 g; Cholesterol: 0 mg; Protein: 1 g; Sodium: 84 mg; Potassium: 391 mg; Fiber: 3 g; Carbohydrates: 13 g; Sugar: 7 g

Cream-style Corn

Servings: 4

Ingredients:

- 1 ½ cups (195 g) frozen corn, cooked, divided
- 2 tablespoons (26 g) sugar

Directions:

1. Place ½ cup (65 g) of the cooked corn, 1/4 cup (60 ml) of the cooking liquid, and the sugar (adjust depending on how sweet you like it) in the blender. Process until mostly liquefied. Add the other cup of corn and process a few seconds at medium speed until kernels are just broken up.

Nutrition Info: (Per Serving): 44 g water; 85 calories (5% from fat, 8% from protein, 87% from carb); 2 g protein; 0 g total fat; 0 g saturated fat; 0 g monounsaturated fat; 0 g polyunsaturated fat; 21 g carb; 2 g fiber; 9 g sugar; 3 mg calcium; 0 mg iron; 3 mg sodium; 181 mg potassium; 150 IU vitamin A; 4 mg vitamin C; 0 mg cholesterol

Steamed Green Beans And Asparagus

Servings: 6

Ingredients:

- 1 pound fresh green beans
- 1 pound fresh asparagus spears
- 3 tablespoons unsalted butter
- 1/3 cup toasted pine nuts
- 1/8 teaspoon white pepper

Directions:

1. Cut both ends off the green beans and rinse well. Bend the asparagus until it snaps, then discard the ends. Rinse well.

2. Bring 1" of water to a simmer in a large saucepan. Put the green beans in a colander or steamer insert and place on top. Cover and steam for 2 minutes.

3. Carefully remove the cover and add the asparagus; mix with the green beans using tongs. Cover again and steam for 2–3 minutes or until the vegetables are bright green and crisp-tender.

4. Transfer vegetables to a serving dish and toss with the butter. Sprinkle with pine nuts and pepper and serve.

Nutrition Info: (Per Serving):Calories: 172; Total Fat: 11 g; Saturated Fat: 4 g; Cholesterol: 15 mg; Protein: 4 g; Sodium: 3 mg; Potassium: 309 mg; Fiber: 4 g; Carbohydrates: 9 g; Sugar: 2 g

Curried Fresh Vegetables

Servings: 4

Ingredients:

- 3 cups (540 g) tomatoes, chopped
- ½ cup (80 g) onion, coarsely chopped
- 1 cup zucchini, cubed
- ½ cup (60 g) green bell pepper, coarsely chopped
- ¼ teaspoon garlic powder
- 1 tablespoon (6.3 g) curry powder

Directions:

1. Combine all ingredients in a saucepan. Cook and stir until vegetables are softened.

Nutrition Info: (Per Serving): 161 g water; 41 calories (10% from fat, 15% from protein, 75% from carb); 2 g protein; 1 g total fat; 0 g saturated fat; 0 g monounsaturated fat; 0 g polyunsaturated fat; 9 g carb; 3 g fiber; 5 g sugar; 29 mg calcium; 1 mg iron; 10 mg sodium; 417 mg potassium; 1043 IU vitamin A; 28 mg vitamin C; 0 mg cholesterol

Citrus-glazed Carrots

Servings: 6

Ingredients:

- 13/4 pounds large peeled carrots, sliced 1/4" thick, or 2 pounds baby carrots
- 1 cup water
- 1/2 cup orange juice
- 1/4 cup lemon juice
- 1/4 cup grapefruit juice
- 3 tablespoons honey
- 2 tablespoons unsalted butter
- 1/2 teaspoon grated orange zest
- 1/2 teaspoon grated lemon zest

Directions:

1. In large pot, combine carrots with water, orange juice, lemon juice, grapefruit juice, and honey. Bring to a boil over high heat.

2. Reduce heat to low and cook, stirring occasionally, until carrots are almost tender, about 5–6 minutes.

3. With a slotted spoon, remove carrots from liquid and set aside.

4.   Boil the remaining liquid in the pot until it is reduced and thickens to a thin syrup.

5.   Return carrots to the liquid along with butter, orange zest, and lemon zest. Simmer for 1–3 minutes or until carrots are glazed and tender. Serve immediately.

Nutrition Info: (Per Serving):Calories: 102; Total Fat: 0 g; Saturated Fat: 0 g; Cholesterol: 0 mg; Protein: 1 g; Sodium: 92 mg; Potassium: 498 mg; Fiber: 3 g; Carbohydrates: 25 g; Sugar: 17 g

Winter Vegetable Casserole

Servings: 6

Ingredients:

- 12 ounces (340 g) frozen winter veggie mix
- 6 ounces (170 g) frozen brussels sprouts
- 1 cup (235 ml) skim milk
- ½ cup (115 g) sour cream
- 2 tablespoons (16 g) cornstarch
- ½ can (6 ounces, or 170 g) water chestnuts
- 2 ounces (55 g) low sodium cheddar cheese

Directions:

1. Cook vegetables according to package directions. Mix milk, sour cream, and cornstarch until blended. Cook and stir until bubbly and thickened. Stir in vegetables and water chestnuts. Place in 9 × 13-inch (23 × 33-cm) baking dish. Sprinkle with cheese and bake at 350°F (180°C, gas mark 4) until cheese is melted, about 10 minutes.

Nutrition Info: (Per Serving): 126 g water; 155 calories (42% from fat, 18% from protein, 40% from carb); 7 g protein; 7 g total fat; 5 g saturated fat; 2 g monounsaturated fat; 0 g polyunsaturated fat; 16 g carb; 4 g fiber; 2 g sugar; 169 mg calcium; 1 mg iron; 61 mg sodium; 295 mg potassium; 564 IU vitamin A; 15 mg vitamin C; 19 mg cholesterol

Oven-dried Seasoned Tomatoes

Servings: 8

Ingredients:

- 4 plum tomatoes, peeled, seeded, and cut into quarters
- Olive oil spray
- 1/8 teaspoon freshly ground black pepper
- 1/2 teaspoon Pasta Blend

Directions:

1. Preheat oven to 250°F.
2. Put the tomatoes in a medium bowl. Lightly mist with the olives oil spray, toss, and then mist again. Add the pepper and Pasta Blend.
3. Arrange the tomatoes on a baking sheet and bake until somewhat dried, about 21/2–3 hours. Store covered, in the refrigerator up to 4 days, or freeze for longer storage.

Nutrition Info: (Per Serving):Calories: 8; Total Fat: 0 g; Saturated Fat: 0 g; Cholesterol: 0 mg; Protein: 0 g; Sodium: 2 mg; Potassium: 106 mg; Fiber: 0 g; Carbohydrates: 1 g; Sugar: 1 g

Baked Cauliflower Casserole

Servings: 6

Ingredients:

- 1 (13/4-pound) head cauliflower
- 1 teaspoon lemon juice
- 1/8 teaspoon mustard powder
- Olive oil spray
- 2 large eggs, beaten
- 1 teaspoon Sonoran Spice Blend
- 1/4 cup grated Parmesan cheese
- 1/2 cup bread crumbs

Directions:

1. Preheat oven to 375°F.

2. Trim off the outer leaves of the cauliflower. Break the cauliflower apart. Bring a large pot of water to a boil over medium-high heat. Add the lemon juice and mustard powder; stir to mix. Add the cauliflower to the water and blanch for 5 minutes. Remove with a slotted spoon and drain.

3. Spray an ovenproof casserole dish with the olive oil spray. Spread the cauliflower evenly in the casserole dish.

4.   In a small bowl, mix together the eggs, Sonoran Spice Blend, and cheese. Evenly pour the mixture over the top of the cauliflower. Sprinkle the bread crumbs over the top and lightly mist with the olive oil spray. Cover and bake for 15 minutes or until the eggs are set and the cheese is melted.

Nutrition Info: (Per Serving):Calories: 90; Total Fat: 3 g; Saturated Fat: 1 g; Cholesterol: 74 mg; Protein: 6 g; Sodium: 139 mg; Potassium: 225 mg; Fiber: 3 g; Carbohydrates: 9 g; Sugar: 3 g

Grilled Onions

Servings: 4

Ingredients:

- 2 onions
- 2 tablespoons (28 g) unsalted butter
- 2 teaspoons (10 ml) sodium-free beef bouillon
- ½ teaspoon garlic powder

Directions:

1. Peel onions. Slice a small section off of one end of each onion and make a small hole in the center. Fill the center of each onion with 1 teaspoon of bouillon, 1 tablespoon (14 g) butter, and ¼ teaspoon garlic powder. Replace the top of the onion and wrap in aluminum foil. Place onions on preheated medium grill and close grill. Cook for 1 hour, or until tender. Cut into bite-size chunks and place In a serving dish with all the juices from the foil.

Nutrition Info: (Per Serving): 55 g water; 79 calories (63% from fat, 4% from protein, 33% from carb); 1 g protein; 6 g total fat; 4 g saturated fat; 2 g monounsaturated fat; 0 g polyunsaturated fat; 7 g

carb; 1 g fiber; 3 g sugar; 16 mg calcium; 0 mg iron; 44 mg sodium; 105 mg potassium; 205 IU vitamin A; 4 mg vitamin C; 15 mg cholesterol

Baked Sweet Potatoes

Servings: 4

Ingredients:

- 4 sweet potatoes
- ¼ cup (60 g) brown sugar
- 1 teaspoon ground cinnamon

Directions:

1. Scrub potatoes and score the skin with a knife to allow the steam to escape. Bake at 375°F (190°C, gas mark 5) until done, about 45 minutes. Sprinkle with brown sugar and cinnamon.

Nutrition Info: (Per Serving): 121 g water; 168 calories (1% from fat, 5% from protein, 94% from carb); 2 g protein; 0 g total fat; 0 g saturated fat; 0 g monounsaturated fat; 0 g polyunsaturated fat; 41 g carb; 4 g fiber; 22 g sugar; 59 mg calcium; 2 mg iron; 46 mg sodium; 398 mg potassium; 2 IU vitamin A; 19 mg vitamin C; 0 mg cholesterol

Baked Cajun Cauliflower

Servings: 6

Ingredients:

- 1 (13/4-pound) head cauliflower
- 1 teaspoon lemon juice
- 1/8 teaspoon mustard powder
- Olive oil spray
- 1/2–1 teaspoon Cajun Spice Blend

Directions:

1. Preheat oven to 375°F.

2. Trim off the outer leaves of the cauliflower. Cut the base so that the head will sit upright. Bring a large pot of water to a boil over medium-high heat. Add the lemon juice and mustard powder; stir to mix. Add the cauliflower, base down, and blanch for 5 minutes. Remove and drain.

3. Spray a deep ovenproof casserole dish with the olive oil spray. Place the cauliflower base down in the casserole dish. Lightly mist the cauliflower with the olive oil spray. Evenly sprinkle the Cajun Spice Blend over the top of

the cauliflower. Cover and bake for 15
minutes.

Nutrition Info: (Per Serving):Calories: 30; Total Fat: 0
g; Saturated Fat: 0 g; Cholesterol: 0 mg; Protein: 2 g;
Sodium: 19 mg; Potassium: 189 mg; Fiber: 3 g;
Carbohydrates: 5 g; Sugar: 2 g

Fresh Veggie Medley

Servings: 4

Ingredients:

- ½ pound (225 g) green beans
- 4 tomatoes, chopped
- 1 zucchini, cubed
- ¼ teaspoon garlic powder
- 1 teaspoon dried basil

Directions:

1. Wash, trim, and cook beans until almost tender. Drain. Return to pan with other ingredients and cook to desired doneness.

Nutrition Info: (Per Serving): 51 g water; 19 calories (3% from fat, 20% from protein, 77% from carb); 1 g protein; 0 g total fat; 0 g saturated fat; 0 g monounsaturated fat; 0 g polyunsaturated fat; 4 g carb; 2 g fiber; 1 g sugar; 25 mg calcium; 1 mg iron; 4 mg sodium; 126 mg potassium; 408 IU vitamin A; 9 mg vitamin C; 0 mg cholesterol

Caribbean Corn On The Cob

Servings: 4

Ingredients:

- 4 cups water
- 1/8 cup lime juice
- 1 teaspoon Caribbean Spice Blend
- 4 medium-size ears yellow sweet corn
- Optional: Freshly ground black pepper

Directions:

1. In a large, deep nonstick sauté pan, bring the water to a boil. Stir in the lime juice and the Caribbean spice blend. Add the corn. Cover, reduce heat, and simmer for 4–6 minutes, until the corn is just tender. Remove corn from pan using tongs and drain briefly. Serve topped with freshly ground black pepper, if desired.

Nutrition Info: (Per Serving):Calories: 61; Total Fat: 0 g; Saturated Fat: 0 g; Cholesterol: 0 mg; Protein: 1 g; Sodium: 2 mg; Potassium: 166 mg; Fiber: 1 g; Carbohydrates: 14 g; Sugar: 0 g

Oriental Vegetable Toss

Servings: 6

Ingredients:

- ½ pound (225 g) lettuce, shredded
- 4 ounces (115 g) snow peas
- ½ cup (65 g) carrot, sliced
- 1 cup (70 g) cabbage, shredded
- 4 ounces (115 g) mushrooms, sliced
- ½ cup (60 g) red bell pepper, sliced
- 4 ounces (115 g) mung bean sprouts
- For dressing:
- ¼ cup (60 ml) Soy Sauce Substitute
- 2 tablespoons (30 ml) rice vinegar
- 2 tablespoons (30 ml) mirin wine
- ½ teaspoon ground ginger
- 1 tablespoon (8 g) sesame seeds

Directions:

1. Toss salad ingredients. Spoon dressing over.

Nutrition Info: (Per Serving): 122 g water; 39 calories (6% from fat, 24% from protein, 71% from carb); 2 g protein; 0 g total fat; 0 g saturated fat; 0 g monounsaturated fat; 0 g polyunsaturated fat; 7 g carb; 2 g fiber; 4 g sugar; 29 mg calcium; 1 mg iron;

16 mg sodium; 269 mg potassium; 1822 IU vitamin A; 34 mg vitamin C; 0 mg cholesterol

Apple Cranberry Coleslaw

Servings: 8

Ingredients:

- 1 head green cabbage, shredded
- 2 Granny Smith apples, shredded
- 1/4 cup sliced green onions
- 2/3 cup Mayonnaise
- 1/4 cup lemon yogurt
- 1/4 cup apple juice
- 2 tablespoons honey
- 1 tablespoon Mustard
- 1 tablespoon lemon juice
- 1 teaspoon dried thyme leaves
- 2/3 cup dried cranberries

Directions:

1. In large bowl, combine cabbage, apples, and green onions.
2. In small bowl, combine mayonnaise, yogurt, apple juice, honey, mustard, lemon juice, and thyme and mix well.
3. Pour over vegetables in large bowl and toss to coat. Stir in cranberries, cover, and

refrigerate for 1–2 hours before serving to blend flavors.

Nutrition Info: (Per Serving):Calories: 260; Total Fat: 16 g; Saturated Fat: 2 g; Cholesterol: 22 mg; Protein: 3 g; Sodium: 34 mg; Potassium: 343 mg; Fiber: 5 g; Carbohydrates: 29 g; Sugar: 21 g

Confetti Corn

Servings: 6

Ingredients:

- 2 tablespoons unsalted butter
- 1 medium red bell pepper, chopped
- 1 medium green bell pepper, chopped
- 1/4 cup sliced green onions
- 1 clove garlic, minced
- 1 (16-ounce) package frozen white and yellow corn, thawed
- 1 cup seeded and chopped tomato
- 1/2 cup heavy cream
- 1/2 teaspoon dried basil leaves
- 1/8 teaspoon black pepper

Directions:

1.   In large saucepan, melt butter over medium heat. Add red bell pepper, green bell pepper, green onions, and garlic; cook and stir until crisp-tender, about 4 minutes.

2.   Add corn and tomato to saucepan; cook and stir until hot, about 2 minutes longer. Add cream, basil, and pepper and bring to a

simmer. Simmer for 1–2 minutes or until slightly thickened. Serve immediately.

Nutrition Info: (Per Serving):Calories: 180; Total Fat: 11 g; Saturated Fat: 7 g; Cholesterol: 37 mg; Protein: 3 g; Sodium: 15 mg; Potassium: 291 mg; Fiber: 3 g; Carbohydrates: 19 g; Sugar: 4 g

Creamy Brown Rice Pilaf

Servings: 4

Ingredients:

- 2 tablespoons unsalted butter
- 1 medium onion, finely chopped
- 3 cloves garlic, minced
- 2 medium carrots, diced
- 1/2 cup diced mushrooms
- 11/3 cups brown rice
- 2 cups Vegetable Broth
- 2/3 cup water
- 1 tablespoon lemon juice
- 1 teaspoon dried marjoram leaves
- 1/2 cup plain yogurt
- 1/3 cup sour cream
- 1/8 teaspoon white pepper

Directions:

1. In a large saucepan, melt butter over medium heat. Add onion, garlic, and carrots; cook, stirring occasionally, until tender. Add mushrooms; cook and stir for another 5 minutes.

2. Add rice; cook and stir for 2 minutes. Then add broth, water, lemon juice, and marjoram; bring to a simmer.

3. Reduce heat to low, cover pan, and simmer for 30–35 minutes or until rice is tender.

4. Remove from heat and stir in yogurt, sour cream, and pepper.

Nutrition Info: (Per Serving):Calories: 393; Total Fat: 13 g; Saturated Fat: 7 g; Cholesterol: 29 mg; Protein: 9 g; Sodium: 95 mg; Potassium: 521 mg; Fiber: 5 g; Carbohydrates: 60 g; Sugar: 4 g

Grilled Corn With Honey Butter

Servings: 6

Ingredients:

- 6 ears corn
- 1/4 cup honey
- 1/4 cup unsalted butter
- 1/8 teaspoon cinnamon

Directions:

1. Prepare and preheat grill. While the grill is preheating, pull back all the leaves on the corn cobs. Remove the silk. Smooth half of the leaves back over the corn kernels; tear off and discard the outer leaves.

2. In small bowl, combine honey, butter, and cinnamon. Mix well and set aside.

3. Grill the corn 6" from medium coals for 15–20 minutes, turning frequently, until the leaves look scorched. Use a kitchen towel to peel off the remaining leaves and serve immediately with honey butter.

Nutrition Info: (Per Serving):Calories: 169; Total Fat: 8 g; Saturated Fat: 4 g; Cholesterol: 20 mg; Protein: 2

g; Sodium: 4 mg; Potassium: 168 mg; Fiber: 2 g; Carbohydrates: 25 g; Sugar: 13 g